Hit It Hard With HIIT!

I0417343

How to Melt Fat And Optimize Performance With High Intensity Interval Training (HIIT) Workouts

RON KNESS

No part of this book may be reproduced, stored in a retrieval system, or transmitted in any form or by any means, electronic, mechanical, photocopying, recording, scanning, or otherwise, without the prior written permission of the publisher, except for the inclusion of brief quotations in a review.

This book is for **personal use only**.

Copyright © 2017 Ron Kness

All rights reserved.

ISBN-13: 978-1544931807

ISBN-10: 1544931808

Contents

Disclaimer

This publication is for informational purposes only and is not intended as medical advice. Medical advice should always be obtained from a qualified medical professional for any health conditions or symptoms associated with them.

Every possible effort has been made in preparing and researching this material. We make no warranties with respect to the accuracy, applicability of its contents or any omissions.

See your healthcare professional before starting any diet, health or exercise program!

Introduction

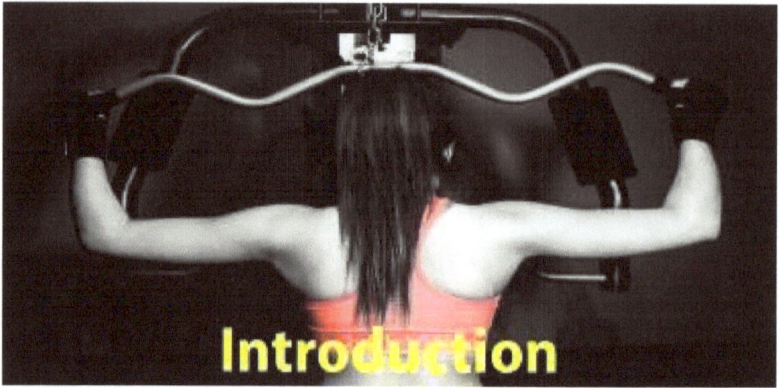

Introduction

Think working out has to be hard? Think again! HIIT workouts appear to do the impossible by helping you to burn more calories than a 40-minute run in a quarter of that time!

Better yet, they also build muscle, improve athletic performance and give you more energy. They've been transforming the lives of people all around the world and if you want to achieve one of those 'cover model physiques' then this is probably just what you're looking for.

Ready to get started with the most highly effective and efficient workouts on the planet? Then let's go! Along the way, we'll discover that there's a lot more to HIIT than just the basic alternating speeds; we'll learn some advanced techniques like cardio acceleration, fartlek training, speed drills, concurrent training, MetCon, Tabata, finishers and more.

Chapter 1: Cardio Training, Then and Now

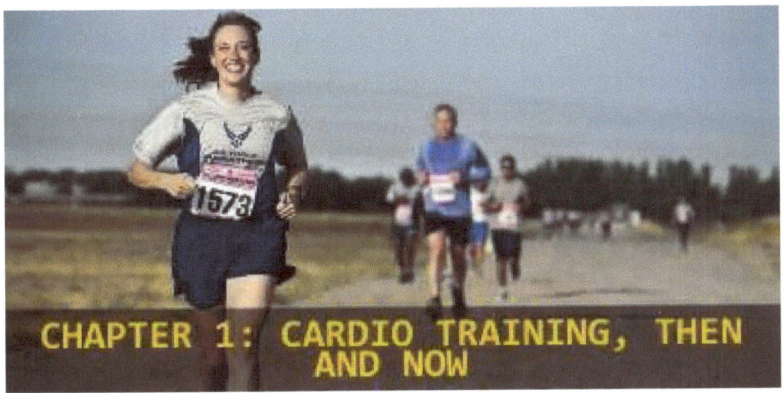

If you want to build muscle, then you need to cause muscle damage and metabolic stress. By lifting weights, you can cause a build-up of damage and this will provide precisely the stimulation you need to trigger muscle growth during rest.

To lose fat, improve your fitness and get better health though, you need to use cardiovascular training.

Cardiovascular training is any type of training that involves exerting yourself for an extended period of time. Very often this will mean running long distances, with jogging being perhaps the most popular form of cardio training. Not far behind though are swimming, cycling, jump rope skipping, rowing and others.

Traditionally, this kind of cardiovascular training has been 'steady state'. That means that you put on your running shoes, you step out of the door and you run *at about the same speed* for about 40-60 minutes.

It's steady state because you are maintaining a steady level of exertion throughout the course of the exercise. In this case you are jogging at a set pace and then maintaining that pace.

For a long time, this was thought to be the very best way to burn the maximum number of calories and to improve fitness – and there was good theory behind why this should be the case. Specifically, it was thought that there was an optimal 'fat burning zone' and that this could be found at roughly 70% of your maximum heartrate.

This makes sense in theory, seeing as faster than 70% of your MHR would put you past your 'anaerobic threshold'. In other words, you would be running so fast, that you wouldn't be able to rely on your aerobic energy system for fuel: you simply couldn't burn fat quickly enough and so you would be forced to rely on energy stored in your muscles as ATP and glycogen.

It would appear to make sense then, that running at 70% of your MHR and maintaining the maximum pace at which the body burns fat, should result in the maximum weight loss.

But this isn't what modern research has found.

HIIT stands for 'High Intensity Interval Training' and it completely turns this concept on its head. In HIIT you actually alternate between bursts of intense exertion (such as sprinting) and periods of relative low intensity exercise (like jogging or power walking). This way, you are switching from your anaerobic energy system to your aerobic system and back; switching between burning energy stored in your blood and muscles and energy stored as fat.

But what makes this so effective is what happens *after* the anaerobic training. When you exert yourself maximally by sprinting or exercising otherwise at 100%, you deplete any energy that might have been available from sources other than fat. This then means that following that, your body can *only* burn fat for energy – there is no other option remaining.

Thus, the you will then burn even more fat during the aerobic portions of the exercise. And when you finish and go home, you will continue to burn fat stores because you'll still be low on stored glycogen. This is what some people refer to as the 'after burn effect' and it means that after an intensive session of HIIT, you can continue to burn more calories for the entire remainder of the day!

More Benefits of HIIT

HIIT is able to burn more calories than steady state cardio then and because you're exerting yourself more at certain

points throughout your training, this means you should also see be finished in a much shorter space of time.

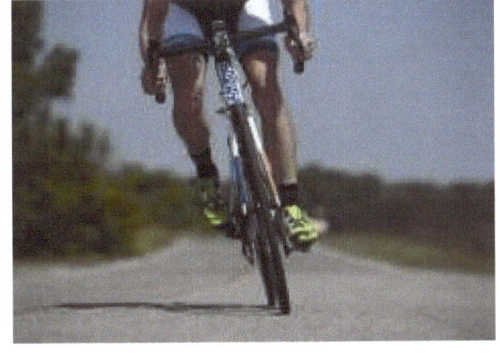

Typically, a HIIT session can last between 10-20 minutes and be just as effective in terms of calories burned as a 40-minute run. For those who have a busy and hectic work schedule then, HIIT training is the ideal solution and allow them to squeeze in a few short minutes of highly effective training to get amazing results!

There are more reasons to get excited about HIIT too.

When looking at any type of training program, what's always useful to keep in mind is the SAID principle. This means 'Specific Adaptations to Imposed Demands' – it means that your body changes to adapt to the demands placed on it.

If you train at altitude, you become better at training at altitude. If you jog, you become better at jogging.

Thus, HIIT makes you better at high intensity activities – which include sprinting, running, rowing, boxing, wrestling, play fighting, sports, moving furniture and more. These are things we are much more likely to utilize in our daily lives and that makes this a more adaptive and useful form of training. Whereas steady state cardio makes you more effective at 'long slogs', HIIT makes you explosive and athletic.

And this also creates a number of other great advantages too. For instance, HIIT has been shown to help improve the efficiency and number of mitochondria. Mitochondria are tiny 'energy factories' that live inside all of our cells and have the critical role of creating and utilizing ATP (adenosine triphosphate). This is the most fundamental form of energy in the human body and it's what fuels all our movements as well as all our thoughts. More mitochondria means greater energy efficiency. That means yet more athletic performance and even more *brain power*. Your brain cells have mitochondria too!

Ever wondered why little kids seem to run in circles all day without getting tired while older generations get exhausted from getting up to turn the TV on?

One of the big reasons for this discrepancy is the difference in the number and efficiency of mitochondria.

This also improves your 'VO2 max', which is the amount of oxygen you are capable of using. The greater your VO2 max, the more efficient you become at oxygenating your body.

This is one of the biggest indicators of physical fitness and one of the things that athletes are encouraged to focus on in their training.

But perhaps best of all is that the kind of explosive movement used in HIIT will invariably engage your 'fast twitch muscle fiber'. These are the muscle fibers that contain more mitochondria and that are responsible for delivering rapid power. They're also the biggest type of muscle fibers and the ones that will make you look like a bodybuilder.

If you engage in steady state cardio, then you can risk converting your fast twitch muscle fiber into slow twitch fiber. Why? Because you are placing high energy demands on your body over a long duration – and thus your body will want to move the ratio toward the most efficient form of muscle fiber. What's more, is that you create a highly catabolic environment that in short starves your body of fuel and forces it to break down both fat *and* muscle.

This is why most long-distance runners also happen to be stick thin.

But when you engage your fast twitch muscle fibers, you show your body that you need explosiveness and you shorten the length of the catabolic period.

This in turn means that you don't risk breaking down muscle tissue in the same way, allowing you to create a physique that is hard, ripped and powerful. Women can expect toned definition, while men can expect rippling vascularity and striations.

That's why, as we stated earlier, this is the preferred weight loss strategy of cover models and celebrities.

So let's recap: this is a form of training that is:

- Quicker than conventional steady state cardio

- Able to burn a much greater number of calories in a shorter time

- Able to create an 'afterburn effect' for increased metabolism throughout the day

- Effective in increasing energy levels by improving the number of mitochondria

- Effective in protecting muscle against deterioration for a leaner, harder physique

- Excellent for your all-round health

Oh and did we mention that it's also highly versatile and practical and can be performed anywhere?

Yep, that's pretty much why people love HIIT. Let's introduce it into your routine, shall we?

Just before we do that though, let's take a closer look at the science. Boring I know – but it will be crucial in helping you to really understand what you're doing, rather than just following a routine blindly!

Chapter 2: The Science of HIIT, Understanding Your Body So You Can Get More Out of It

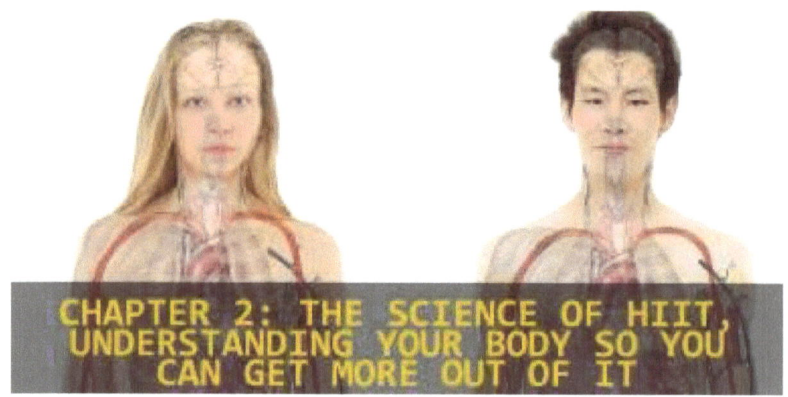

Let's first consider how the body gets energy and manages that energy during exertion.

First, in order to exercise, the body needs energy. This energy comes from a source known as ATP or Adenosine Triphosphate which is described in scientific circles as the 'energy currency of life'. This substance is a nucleotide made up of three phosphagen molecules, bonded together by a powerful force. That's what the name literally means tri- meaning three, phosphate – meaning phosphagen.

All types of energy in the body are ultimately converted into ATP, so when you eat a big cake, the sugar and glucose will ultimately need to be converted into this molecule before it can be of any use to your muscles or your cells. In real terms, any one 'mole' of ATP energy will provide 7.3 calories. It would take just over 190 micromoles to move your index finger enough to click a mouse button on a computer and this would equate to around 1.42 calories!

The power in this substance however doesn't come from the phosphagen itself, but from the powerful bonds that bind it together, and it's when these bonds break that they unleash the energy that the body can utilize. An athlete needs to be able to supply their muscles with a lot of ATP then in order to perform the necessary movements for running or weightlifting – and there are three ways in which they can do this.

The Three Energy Systems

The first way the body gets ATP is through the phosphagen system, also known as the ATP-CP system, which uses the ATP stored in the muscles to supply that energy. The body can store enough ATP at any one time to allow for around 3 seconds of full powered exertion (a little more or a little less depending on your physical fitness and various other factors), at which point it will need to look elsewhere.

Fortunately breaking the ATP molecules results in some useful bi products – ADP (andenosinediphosphate) and AMP (andenosine monophosphate) with two and one bonded phosphagen molecules respectively. So if you imagine you have three bonded molecules and they break you will understandably be left with a one and a two, or three single molecules. It's basic math... The good news is that using a substance called creatine phosphate (hence the CP!) can then recombine these molecules to make them back into ATP ready to be broken once more for extra energy. The body can store enough creatine for roughly 8-10 seconds of continued exertion, meaning that in total the body can use the phosphagen system for around 13 seconds maximum of continued exertion. That is enough to sprint just over 100 meters.

It is thought however that through the use of creatine supplements that this maximum time can be increased marginally.

At this point if exertion continues the body needs to get its ATP from somewhere else and this is when it looks to its stored carbohydrates in the form of glycogen. This represents the shift to what is known as the 'glycogen lactic acid system'.

This system is a slightly slower and less efficient means of supplying energy, which requires the body to split the glycogen first into glucose and then again into ATP. This unfortunately creates a number of unwanted by-products called metabolites including lactic acid (from which the substance takes its name).This metabolic build-up creates the uncomfortable, mildly painful 'burning' sensation we get in our muscles when we push ourselves in the gym. The body can sustain itself using the glycogen lactic acid system for a further one minute and thirty seconds until this build up becomes too much to tolerate. If we continue to try and push ourselves at MHR past this point, it can lead to nausea and even fainting.

It was long believed that lactic acid was actually responsible for this failure and for the burning sensation. However, more recent research has shown us that lactate is not harmful in itself but rather seems to correlate with other factors that fatigue the glycogen lactic acid system. Thus high level athletes can still monitor their build-up of lactate in the blood in order to calculate a 'lactate inflection point'. With training, it is possible to improve tolerance to metabolites and thus sustain maximum exertion for longer.

Guess what you can use to improve this aspect of your fitness? HIIT!

Both these systems are anaerobic, meaning that for the first one minute and forty-three seconds the body won't be using oxygen or burning fat.

In order to lose weight then the training must continue past this point and force the body to find its energy elsewhere. This is where the aerobic system comes in, relying on the oxidization of foodstuffs in our mitochondria. In other words, the body looks to our supplies of glycogen (and ATP) stored in our cells as fat and then uses the oxygen in our blood to break them down and carry them to our muscles. This is then what leads to fat being burned directly. This forces us to breathe more heavily in order to supply the necessary amount of oxygen and it increase our heartrate further to transport the oxygen to the fat stores and then to bring the energy to our muscles and brain.

The aerobic energy system can actually be used indefinitely and will continue until you completely exhaust all supplies of energy located around the body. During a typical prolonged endurance test, you will find you also breakdown protein for energy and even muscle. This in contrast to high intensity exercises that will use 100% carbohydrates for fuel, purely because they provide the quickest and most accessible source of ATP.

How We Progress Through Energy Systems

So if you head outside and start jogging, you'll notice that at first, you don't need to gasp for breath in order to maintain your speed and your heartrate doesn't immediately go crazy. That's because you are using your ATP-CP system.

If you continue this exertion though, you will switch to your glycogen lactic acid system. This will use up energy stored as glycogen in the muscles. This will lead to an increase in lactate and metabolites in the muscles and the blood stream, leading to nausea, muscle pain, cramping and more. It's at this point that things become uncomfortable.

If you are running fast, you will continue to use this system until you eventually pass out – this is your 'lactate threshold' or your 'lactate inflection point'. This is the point at which the build-up of lactate and metabolites becomes too great for you to maintain that level of exercise. This will happen before you have completely exhausted the stored glycogen in the muscles.

But most of us will instead find we are forced to slow down before we reach our inflection point and switch to the aerobic system. We'll drop to sub-maximal exertion triggered by the physical symptoms and will find a steady pace at around 70% of our maximum heartrate. This will mean we have time to burn fat for fuel, which will require heavy breathing and a high heartrate but which won't lead to the same levels of discomfort.

If you were training with steady state cardio, you would continue this level of exertion indefinitely and stop after you'd burned a satisfactory number of calories. Following this, your body would then continue to use a combination of all three systems for tasks throughout the remainder of the day. Low blood sugar however would trigger a release of the hunger hormone ghrelin and this would be accompanied by cortisol (the stress hormone). This is why we're always stressed when we're hungry!

This would also correlate with an increase in myostatin – an unpopular molecule that leads to an increased breakdown of muscle. This is on top of the increased protein breakdown during the exercise itself.

But if you utilize HIIT, you will use the aerobic system for a set period of time giving your body enough time to clear the lactate build-up in your bloodstream and then you would switch *back* to maximum exertion to further deplete the glucose stores. This would mean you were taking a small break from burning fat and blood sugar thus reducing the negative impact on your mood and muscle mass. Moreover, it would mean you could almost entirely empty your glycogen stores and thereby force your body to use blood sugar and fat stores for even the simplest movements for a long period afterward while it creates more glycogen!

Chapter 3: How to Start HIIT Training With Running

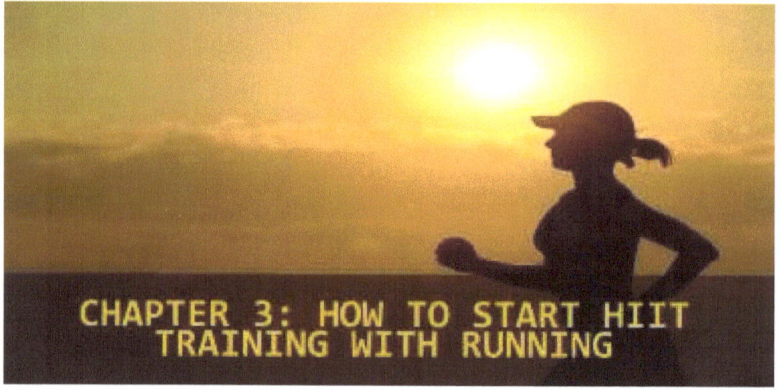

So now you know the science, it's time to start putting that theory into practice!

The great news is that HIIT training really is *just* as easy as it sounds and simply involves alternating between periods of high exertion and relatively low intensity exercise. There are a few caveats however and it is important to approach this in a sensible and structured way in order to avoid injury or disappointment.

Most people will begin their HIIT with running as this is a very straightforward form of cardio training that doesn't require access to any specialist tools and that anyone can understand and use.

There are countless HIIT protocols however, and these vary in length and intensity. The key thing to recognize here is that high intensity training of *any kind* can be highly dangerous if you have never done it before, if you're very overweight or if you're in very poor physical health.

It's also dangerous if you have any pre-existing heart conditions.

In short, you need basic heart strength before you start pushing it to 100%. Thus, it is a good idea to build up at least a basic level of fitness before you start your HIIT training. If you're still gasping for breath whenever you ascend the stairs, then you're not ready for HIIT.

But here's the thing: even if you're used to exercising regularly and you're in good shape, switching to HIIT will still come as a very big shock if you've not used it before. This is a whole new ball game in terms of the demands it places on your body and you'll be surprised at how quickly you end up in a gasping heap on the floor!

If you've never exercised before, then read the next section. If you've not used HIIT before but you're generally in good shape, then you can skip to the one after it.

How to Build Up a Basic Level of Fitness

Note: Before beginning an intensive training routine, it is *always* a good idea to consult with your healthcare professional to ensure that you don't have any underlying heart conditions! Or anything else that could be dangerous if you pursue HIIT.

Before you start pushing yourself to your cardiovascular limit, it's a good idea to first build up that basic level of fitness that will prevent you from shocking your heart too much. Right now, you might be thinking that you don't need to worry about this and that it's not likely you're going to suffer heart problems.

Even if you're not worried though, building this basic level of fitness is important for your ability to stick with an intense HIIT workout.

This is the mistake that too many people make – they launch straight into their training and hope that they'll be able to keep up a pace that is far above what they find 'comfortable'. The belief is that you need to be pushing beyond your comfort levels in order to lose weight.

But what actually happens is that you end up hating exercise and dreading your workouts. The result is that you'll find yourself putting it off and unable to take part unless you're feeling your very best. In no time at all, your training falls by the wayside and you give up!

So don't aim to start losing weight or transform your fitness right away. Rather, focus on gradually improving your fitness so that your workouts are never outside the realms of comfortable to begin with. You'll find that as you do this, you learn to 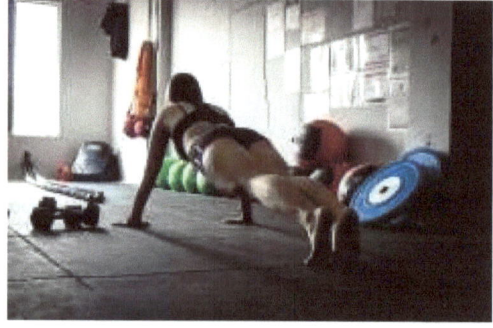 do more and eventually this allows you to take on more challenging workouts and actually stick with them.

So how do you build up this basic fitness?

The answer is actually to start with steady state cardio, using a gentle pace to begin with and then build up. Begin with running but don't aim to run a long distance or to run quickly to begin with. Instead, just aim to *enjoy* running.

Set out with comfortable running shoes and jog carefully and slowly for half an hour. When it becomes painful, go home.

Do this once a week and over time, you'll find that you start running faster and further without even trying. Importantly though, you won't risk exhausting your body, you won't damage your knees, overtraining or learning to loathe your training.

This can be very frustrating at first if you were hoping to get into great shape right away! But what's very important here is to be disciplined with yourself. A lot of people think that getting into great shape is all about being disciplined enough to *keep training*. Just as important though is to be disciplined enough to be patient and to build that basic level of strength before you approach the more intense types of training.

Build up your strength and stamina slowly and *then* you can look at adding HIIT workouts. And again, you're going to start gently...

A Gentle Introduction to HIIT

A lot of people will read the words 'HIIT' and assume that this is one type of workout. In reality though, HIIT is a very broad and flexible term that can encompass a great many different types of training and a great many different protocols.

One of the biggest mistakes you can make then, is to start HIIT and dive in right at the deep end with an intensive program aimed at the incredible fitness One of the most popular choices for instance is Tababta.

This is a brutal, punishing, fast and highly effective method of training that will leave you gasping for air and covered in sweat in just 4 minutes. But it's also far too intense to start with and especially when running.

So instead, let's begin with a very easy beginner routine:

- **Jog for 2 minutes**

- **Sprint for 10 seconds**

Repeat this five times. It sounds very easy but you'll quickly find that just 10 seconds of sprinting is more than enough to completely exhaust you. By the time you're finished, you'll be completely exhausted and you'll feel as though you can't perform another 2 minute jogging session.

Finish with a 10 minute cool down.

The entire workout will take you 12 minutes but you'll find you're easily as tired (if not more tired) than you would have been after jogging at a steady state for 30-40 minutes! Moreover, this is enough to trigger the after-burn effect and to leave you burning calories for hours afterward.

Because this type of training is so fast, you can only afford to do this 2 or 3 times a week. Once you start to become more confident, you can then move on to the next step up:

- **Jog for 2 minutes**

- **Sprint for 30 seconds**

You can also increase the number of laps to 8 and then ten.

Eventually, you might be able to work all the way up to:

- **Jog for 1 minute**

- **Sprint for 30 seconds**

Or

- **Jog for 1 minute**

- **Sprint for 1 minute**

Again though, you should only move on to these harder difficulty levels once you have built up the basic fitness and heart strength to be able to cope relatively easily. You should be exhausted at the end but not to the point where you can't do anything for the rest of the day, or where you're unable to train again for days and days on end.

Chapter 4: Tips for Better HIIT Results

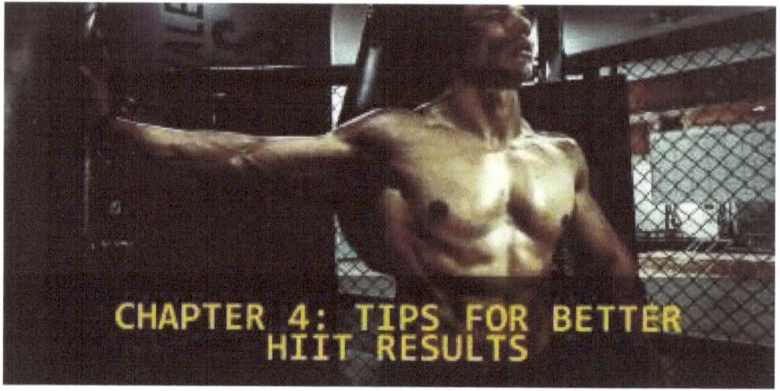

When performing the sprints, remember that it doesn't actually matter how fast you are going as long as you are maxing out your potential. In other words, there's a good chance that you are going to find yourself slowing down somewhat as you reach the later stages of your routine and you shouldn't worry if that happens.

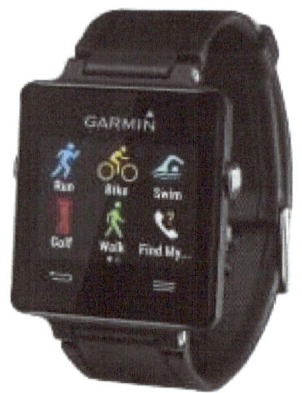

Wearing a fitness tracker or running watch can help you with this. Something like the Garmin Vivoactive (http://amzn.to/2nHir0x) will provide the best of both worlds here by acting as a fitness tracker throughout the day (measuring your heartrate and your steps etc.) but acting as a running watch during training and letting you monitor your route and your metrics.

Your maximum heartrate is something you can calculate quite easily. Simply go for a sprint or engage in other activity with maximum effort. Monitor your heartrate and you should find that it never goes beyond a certain point.

This point is your max heartrate and it's what you should be aiming to hit whenever you perform the high intensity portions of these workouts. The *speed* is less important.

And of course you can also use this to work out 70% of your MHR, which should be your fat burning zone.

Should You Use Machines?

While HIIT itself is fairly simple to grasp, there are actually a lot of different factors to consider.

For example, you need to decide whether to use exercise machines or to avoid them and train outside instead. If you're going to use HIIT for running for instance, should you use a treadmill or should you head outside and jog and sprint?

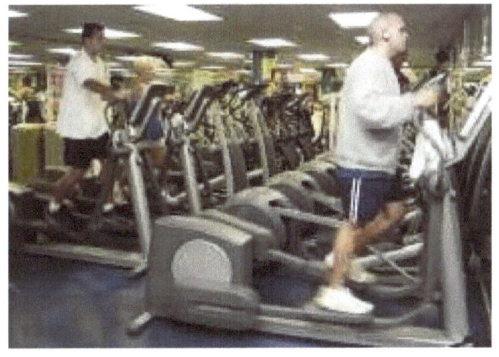

The answer is that it's up to you (of course) and both have their advantages. What's key is to recognize the different benefits of each and therefore to be able to make the best decision for you.

A lot of people will look down on exercise machines. There are indeed a number of problems with these: for starters, they prevent you from getting outside which in itself has a huge number of different health benefits.

At the same time though, you'll also find that running outside has the advantage of training your legs harder and actually uses significantly different biomechanics.

That's because running on a pavement or grass will require pulling force generated in your legs as you have to pull your body along the ground. Wind, elevation, temperature, weather and altitude all affect the amount of energy expended when exercising outside verses inside.

Conversely, when you run on a treadmill, you will only need to lift your legs off the ground as the treadmill moves underneath you. And yes you can adjust the incline and speed, it is still different (and more demanding) exercising outside. As such, there is actually *less* effort involved in running on a treadmill.

Running outside is also a lot more varied. While it's possible to alter the angle and the pace on a treadmill, it's still going to involve selecting from one of a number of different positions and sticking with it. When you run outside meanwhile, you are forced to constantly adapt to changes in the shape of the ground, to the gradient you are running on and more.

Of course many of these issues are less significant if you are riding a stationary bike but the variety and the real world 'value' of running is one of the things that attracts a lot of people to it in the first place.

But this doesn't mean there is no place at all for running on a treadmill. For starters, running on a treadmill is a good option if you have a bad knee or another complaint.

Running at a fixed incline is a good way to reduce the strain on the knees and many people will thus prefer to stick to a treadmill so that they can control this facet. Better yet for bad knees or back complaints is to ride a stationary 'recumbent bike'.

Bikes have zero impact, which makes them better for those with joint complaints. A recumbent bike meanwhile is a type of bike that has you leaning backward with your legs outstretched in front of you. This in turn means that you aren't placing any weight on your legs or your spine and can simply concentrate on driving the pedals.

CV machines are also great for training when you can't be bothered to head outside because it's raining or cold and if you're someone who will struggle to be motivated in this regard, then you should consider that a *very* big bonus. It's *always* better to perform an easier form of exercise and stick with it, than it is to perform a more challenging form but then give up after the first week!

Lastly, running on machines will give you the ability to *precisely* control the level of challenge. That means that you can monitor the exact speed you're able to maintain and a very good estimate of your calorie burn. Some will even include heartrate monitors or synchronize with external gadgets to perform this job. All this is ideal for HIIT because it means you can run for exactly 1 minute at a very precise speed and then switch. Next week, you can do the *exact same thing* and once you're used to that you can increase the challenge by a very small and precise amount.

Incorporating Fasted Cardio

Before we get into the different tools and strategies you can use to mix up your HIIT training, note that there *is* a way you can increase your calorie burn significantly simply by changing the time of day that you train.

This technique is called 'fasted cardio' and it involves training first thing in the morning before breakfast.

This is called 'fasted' cardio because your body is in a fasted state. While you haven't been consciously starving yourself, you will not have eaten for a while merely as a result of having been asleep for so long.

This means that your body will be very low on energy reserves as your glycogen stores and blood sugar are all but depleted. You'll have higher levels of cortisol as a result, which is why many of us are cranky in the morning and it's even one of the things that actually wake us up! Cortisol is one of our 'wakefulness' neurotransmitters and works in direct opposition to melatonin.

If you train at this point then, *before* breakfast, you'll be training at a massive calorie deficit and you'll be forced to burn more fat.

Unfortunately, this also means you're more likely to burn muscle. This is mitigated to some extent by performing HIIT rather than steady state cardio and especially if you are using concurrent training (see below) but it's worth bearing in mind if your goal is to build lean muscle. If your goal is simply weight loss though, then go for it! Just make sure to give yourself a few minutes after getting up so your spine is less vulnerable to injury.

Chapter 5: Concurrent Training and Using Kettlebells

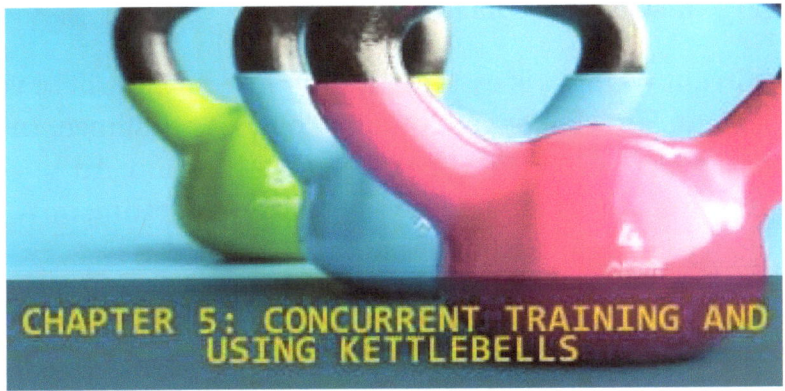

As you begin using HIIT to build basic levels of fitness and progress to improve your metabolism and performance, you can then branch out to try more varied and challenging protocols. What's more, is that many of these types of training can help to provide very specific benefits and help you to reach particular goals. If you know precisely what it is that you're trying to achieve with your training, then you might find that one of these types of training is actually the most advantageous for you...

In this chapter, we're going to be looking at adding an additional layer of resistance into our training. In the next chapter, we'll learn how to mix up the timing in order to alter the challenge.

Concurrent Training (Resistance Cardio)

One of the best ways to mix up your training is to change the type of exercise that you're using in your HIIT routines.

This is something we'll discuss a lot more in the next chapters but the first thing to consider is combining cardio and resistance training together in the form of 'resistance cardio' – also called 'concurrent training'.

Concurrent training is essentially a type of cardio where your movements are challenged by some form of resistance. In short, it's like weightlifting *combined* with cardio. An obvious example is to increase the resistance setting on a stationary bike, or to run on sand.

But actually, there are much better examples. One is to perform pull-ups quickly, or to perform press-ups quickly. You can also try punching a heavy bag (which requires muscle power in the shoulders in particular), or you can try running while pushing or pulling something heavy behind or in front of you.

This has a huge number of advantages, the principle one being that it is even *more* protective against muscle deterioration. That is to say that you can perform this kind of cardio and burn a *lot* of calories without worrying that you'll lose much muscle. This is because you're engaging even more of your fast twitch muscle fibers and you're driving blood and metabolites to your muscles where they will stimulate growth.

At the same time, that increase in growth hormone and testosterone (triggered by the breakdown of muscle) will mean an improved level of fat burning and muscle building. Anabolic hormones such as these don't only encourage the body to build muscle but also to burn fat – which is why steroid users look so incredibly lean as well as being incredibly strong.

Of course steroids also have a ton of very serious side effects, so this is a way that we can get the same kind of anabolic results without the dangers associated with them.

Building muscle at the same time as burning fat will help you to create a much superior physique too and this is something that a lot of people don't realize. If you're unhappy with your current physique right now and you want to look more attractive in and out of your clothes, then simply losing weight will make you either look very skinny or potentially even flabby if you have lots of loose skin left over.

Want to get rid of cellulite? Losing weight won't do it. The *only* way to get rid of it is to tone up your legs, buttocks or whatever the offending area may be.

Want to get a flat stomach? Far from burning fat, the best way to do this is actually to strengthen the 'transverse abdominis' – the muscle that wraps around your mid-section and that is responsible for keeping your organs and your gut 'pulled in'.

The best example of all? The kettlebell swing…

Introducing the Kettlebell Swing

When you look up HIIT protocols, you'll find that it's very common to see them recommended for kettlebell swings. That's because the kettlebell swing is in many ways the ideal choice for HIIT and especially if you're interested in building muscle as well as burning fat. And you'll find in some gyms they use both the kettlebell swing *and* HIIT as part of their favorite tools for their workouts.

To perform a kettlebell swing, you of course need a kettlebell. This is an iron ball that has a handle on the top. You can then lift the ball using the handle and treat it like a dumbbell. Unlike a dumbbell though, a kettlebell has the weight located at the bottom and this moves the center of gravity. Now, as you lift the handle, the position of the weight will change, altering the angle of the resistance. You'll also be able to swing the kettlebell in a variety of ways, which causes that weight to move away and toward you respectively. This now adds an additional challenge, which is coping with the momentum of the kettlebell and avoiding letting it pull or push you off balance.

As a result, the kettlebell uses a lot of smaller supporting muscles that are overlooked in other types of training and this helps you to develop 'functional strength'.

The swinging motion also means that you can use various different forms of continuous motion, which is ideal for all kinds of CV challenges. This is exactly our objective when using the kettlebell swing, where we will be swinging the weight between our legs up and down in a pendulum motion.

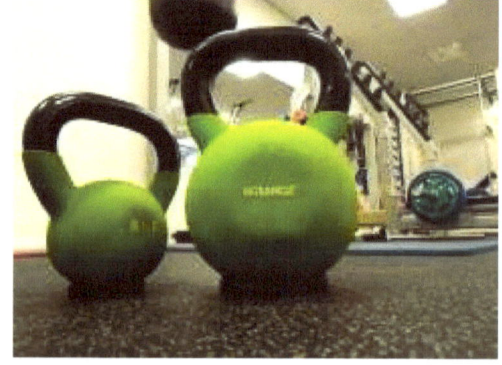

Simply grab the kettlebell in both hands and choose a weight that is going to become challenging after 20 seconds. You should be standing straight with your legs shoulder-width apart and the kettlebell hanging in front of you, held in both hands with arms straight.

Squat down slightly and as you do, allow the kettlebell to swing in between your legs. Now, push through your legs to stand back up and as you do, thrust your hips forward to push the weight out in front of you. Keep your arms straight and don't attempt to 'lift' the weight but instead let it swing up naturally in front of you.

For a traditional kettlebell swing, it should reach about the height of your shoulders (the 'American Swing' reaches above your head).

For a second, the kettlebell will hang in the air and then it will start to descend again as gravity starts to do its thing. Follow the trajectory downward and as you do, drop back into the squat position and let the weight swing back through your legs again. That's one repetition.

Unlike other weighted exercises like curls or bench presses, the kettlebell swing is perfect for cardio exercises because you can keep going and allow gravity to do its thing as you start tiring. Because you're involving your muscles though, you'll find it burns more calories (simply because it is harder than running normally) and you'll protect your muscles from deterioration.

The specific muscles used in the kettlebell swing are all those that make up the 'posterior chain'. These are the muscles in the back and the legs that you use for jumping and for sprinting and thus this is an excellent way to improve your overall athletic performance.

What's more is that these are many of the muscles that we consider most attractive. For women looking to improve their legs, bums and tums, the kettlebell swing is one of the very best choices.

In fact, there is something of an internet meme going around at the moment called 'women who squat'. It's become common knowledge that squatting gives women a *great* behind. The kettlebell swing works all the same muscles but also burns fatting, making it the perfect sculpting tool.

Men who use the exercise meanwhile will benefit from the core involvement and the weight loss that makes it ideal for creating toned abs.

The best bit? The kettlebell is simple, cheap and easy to use. Instead of heading outside in the rain to perform your HIIT workouts, you can use this right at home over the course of 20 minutes.

Chapter 6: Advanced HIIT Protocols – Tabata, MetCon and Cardio Acceleration

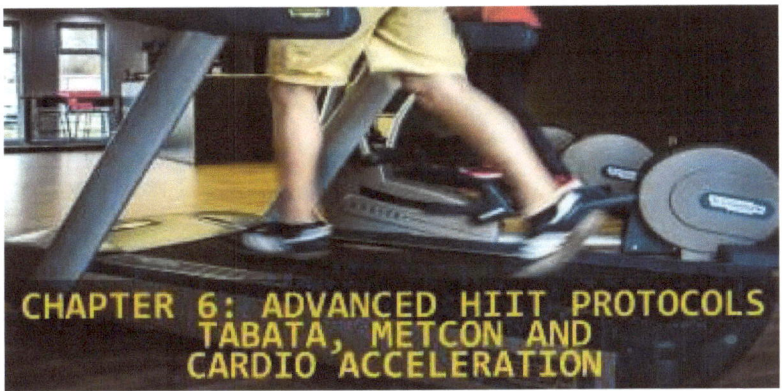

Tabata

We have already mentioned Tabata, which is one of the best known examples of HIIT and one of the most efficient and brutally effective options for burning lots of fat and at the same time toning and building muscle.

The best thing about Tabata? It takes only *four minutes* to get an incredibly intense workout. That's because the split is incredibly short, consisting of:

- **20 seconds of high intensity**

- **10 seconds of rest**

You then repeat the process for a total of 8 times.

Twenty seconds might not sound like a long period of high intensity but when you only have 10 seconds of rest between each burst, you'll find it becomes *incredibly* taxing and that your body will be begging you to stop toward the end. This is ideal because it will train your ability to recover and to remove the lactate and metabolites from your system so that you're ready to return to your first two energy systems to provide fuel.

You can use Tabata for running but actually it is arguably more popular when combined with other exercises such as those 'resistance cardio' methods we discussed in the last chapter. Grab a 30kg (about 66 pounds) kettlebell and perform Tabata using that and you'll be absolutely exhausted by the end and should be able to feel your heart racing in your chest. Another good option is to use some form of jumping exercise – such as jack in the boxes or tuck jumps. You can even vary it up by creating a circuit that allows you to go from one exercise to another. We'll look at this more in subsequent chapters.

Note that if you find Tabata too punishing to begin with, you can perform fewer repetitions – 4 circuits of Tabata is more than hard enough but doesn't have the unwanted side effect of making your heart burst out through your rib cage.

Tabata is a strange way of training because it will tax you incredibly in a short space of time but isn't particularly effective on its own for weight loss or body transformations due to its brevity.

A solution is to use Tabata as what is known as a 'finisher'. A finisher is a type of workout you do at the end of another workout, so if you have completed a weight lifting session or perhaps a session of regular steady state cardio, then you can incorporate Tabata at the end to finish off and thereby maximize your calorie burn for the rest of the day while depleting any and all remaining glycogen stores.

Note as well that Tabata is unique from the HIIT workouts we've looked at so far in as much as it has a real 'rest period' rather than a period of lighter activity. You can swap this for 'active recovery' if you prefer and do that by holding plank for example, or by jogging very lightly on the spot.

A Side Note

A side note that applies to Tabata in particular but to all these HIIT workouts to a degree is just how powerful this is for training your mental discipline. When you're absolutely exhausted, pushing yourself to the absolute limit *again* can be incredibly hard. This requires a lot of mental discipline and self-control and that is actually one of the things that is most exciting and beneficial about HIIT in general.

If you can complete a punishing round of Tabata... then you can complete anything!

Cardio Acceleration

Finding Tabata too easy? Want more of a challenge?

What is *wrong* with you?

As it happens though, if you're that sadistic, then I do just so happen to have something even worse up my sleeve and this is also a great choice if you're someone who is interested in building muscle and creating a *really* ripped physique.

Say hello to 'cardio acceleration'...

Essentially, cardio acceleration is a perversion of HIIT and of resistance training that combines a full gym workout with a cardio workout.

Normally, if you are working out in the gym in order to build muscle, you will do so by performing exercises as 'reps and sets'. You perform a 'set' of 6, 8, 10 or 12 exercises and then you rest for a minute before going again.

What you are doing in this case is building up metabolites in the muscle that stimulate growth and creating microtears.

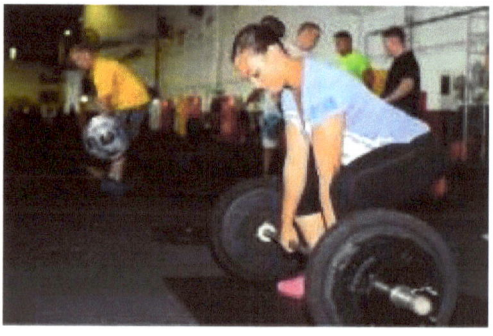

The heavy weight means that you're using your fastest twitch muscle fiber, which means that you'll be relying on glycogen and ATP stored in the muscle. You thus need to pause after performing those 10 reps in order to build up the strength to go again for the next round.

The most common protocol for the gym is to perform 3 sets of 10 reps on each exercise.

Cardio acceleration turns this into a monstrosity of a challenge though by removing the minute rest in between each exercise.

You're still going to give the muscle a rest but you're no longer going to give your body a rest because you're going to perform some kind of cardio exercise such as tuck jumps, high knees, sprinting, step machine, skipping etc. And you'll do this with high intensity.

What you'll also do, is to target the muscles that you *aren't* using. So if you just performed bench press, then you won't use boxing as your cardio to pair it with because that will train the pecs and shoulders again. Likewise, if you just did squats, you're not going to train with kettlebell swings or tuck jumps.

Cardio acceleration works absolute wonders for your body because it allows you to get all the benefits of a weightlifting workout *and* all the benefits of a cardio workout rolled into one. That means that you will build muscle, while at the same time burning fat.

What's more, is that you'll be able to keep your heartrate high for your entire weightlifting routine. This means that you'll burn an incredible number of calories and specifically several hundred percent *more*.

Because you're training the upper body and lower body intermittently, this also has the advantage of directing blood from top to bottom. In other words, you'll need plenty of oxygen and nutrients in your biceps for those curls and then you'll need them in your legs for that sprinting. Thus your heart is working even harder to send the blood up and down and up and down and you'll burn even *more* calories.

The hormonal response to this kind of training is also massive.

There are downsides too though of course. The first is that cardio acceleration is absolutely horrendous to go through. This is a serious challenge and should only be attempted once you're very fit *and* very strong already. It's also something you probably won't want to do very regularly.

The other downside is that you won't build as much muscle as you would do from a regular weightlifting workout. That's because you'll be depleting your strength and thus won't be able to perform your lifts with as much weight or as good technique.

If your aim is to become a massive bodybuilder-type, then you should stay away from cardio acceleration. However, if your aim is to become a lean machine who would look incredible on the cover of a fitness magazine, then you should think about it.

Just be ready for a real challenge!

Fartlek

Fartlek may just be the most ridiculous sounding name for a workout but it's actually a very useful tool so let's not judge this particularly rose by its name!

In fact, fartlek actually translates directly as 'time play'. It is so called because you are going to be dividing your regular cardio workouts in a manner of ways to suit your particular training goals. This way, you can combine steady state cardio with interval training and build towards a variety of different objectives at once.

To explain it simply, fartlek merely means that you can choose how you want to divide your time between sprinting, jogging, walking and everything in between. And it doesn't just have to be time that is the deciding factor here either – you can just as easily train so that you switch speed depending on the distance, or so that you watch your heart rate.

For example, a great way to improve your recovery times is to sprint for 1 minute and then jog gradually *until* your heart rate reaches 70% of your MHR again. When that happens, you increase your speed once more and then go slow until it is back at 70%.

Another interesting challenge is to introduce more outside factors to make things more exciting and less predictable. For instance, keep an eye on the street lamps you are passing. Each time you go past one, change your speed until the next one. You might sprint, jog, walk, sprint, jog, walk – or find another way to switch things up. The same thing can be achieved with a skipping rope or kettlebell.

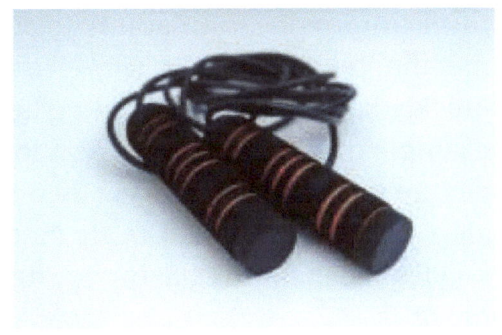

Alternatively, you can try to jog for distance and then sprint at the end to burn off the remaining calories and improve your lactate threshold, *etc.*

Finally, one I find particularly enjoyable is something I call 'anabolic running'. Here, you simply sprint 100 meters, walk back and then sprint the distance again.

This also has the advantage of letting you perform a very intensive cardio workout without needing to travel a long distance – because you don't always have the luxury of being near a beautiful scenic park and sometimes you need to stay close to home.

MetCon

MetCon is a portmanteau for the words 'Metabolic' and 'Conditioning'. As this might suggest then, MetCon is a form of workout that is designed specifically with the goal of helping you to strengthen your metabolism in order to improve your energy efficiency, resting metabolic rate and generally your ability to turn food into useable energy.

The aforementioned fartlek example that challenges you to start running again each time your heartrate reaches 70% can also be considered an example of MetCon for instance, as this is improving your ability to clear your blood of metabolites and lactate, as well as your ability to recover quickly back to a steady resting heartrate. This is a good example of MetCon as well as a form of 'zone training'. If you get the right fitness tracker, then this can actually be used to alert you once your heart rate reaches specific zones – saving you from constantly having to check your wrist every minute or so!

More often though, the term MetCon is used to describe short, focused bursts of high intensity activity with a minimum amount of rest in between. A good example is the 'ladder workout' which involves performing 10 good reps of a given exercise (such as pull-ups, or clapping exercises), resting for 30 seconds and then performing 9 reps. You keep going until you reach 1 repetition, at which point the challenge has ended.

The circuit routines we'll look at in the next chapter can also be considered examples of MetCon.

Chapter 7: Creating Whole-Body Circuit Routines

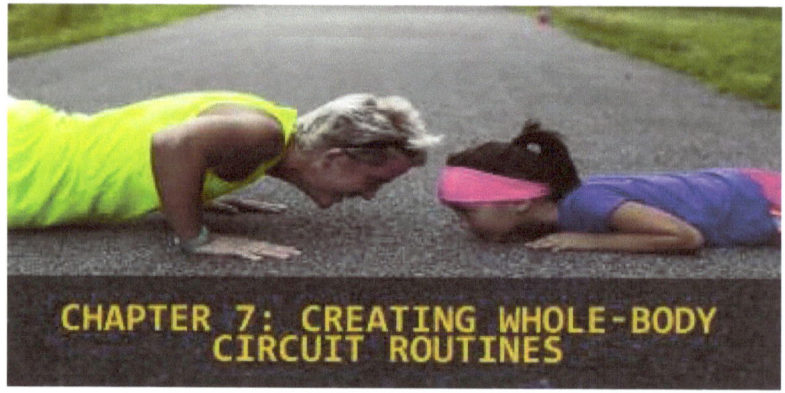

If you look for a workout on YouTube, then you'll find there is no shortage of content available to help out. In particular, you'll find a lot of videos from the likes of Mike Chang (*https://www.youtube.com/results?search_query=mike+chang*), Jeff Cavaliere (*https://www.youtube.com/results?search_query=Jeff+Cavaliere+*) and other YouTube celebrities that promise you can get great results in 20 minutes by following along.

Invariably, these workouts will essentially boil down to circuit routines. They will set up a few stations in a small space and then they will train on each one for a set amount of time before moving to the next.

This circuit training is a very simple way of working out that has been around *forever* but it is also something that has come back into vogue in a big way since HIIT became so popular. That's partly due to their similarities and with a renewed understanding of what makes HIIT so effective, we're keen to apply these same ideas to other types of workout.

Circuit training like this can thereby be designed to work as a form of MetCon while also offering resistance cardio (concurrent training) and being very easy to perform in a small amount of space and short amount of time.

But just because circuit training has the potential to be highly effective, that certainly doesn't mean it always is! In fact, circuit training can very often be a waste of time – and especially if you watch the wrong channel! (Not *all* of Six Pack Shortcut's workouts are that well thought out for example...).

There is an art to designing the perfect circuit and getting this right will depend partly on your goals...

How to Design the Perfect Circuit Routine

The first thing to consider before you begin your circuit plan, is exactly what it is you hope to achieve through it.

As you're reading a book on HIIT, chances are that you want to burn calories and lose fat in a short amount of time and essentially turn this into a form of HIIT or MetCon. The problem is that a lot of circuits just don't offer enough of a challenge for your cardiovascular system for you to accomplish this. If your workout is made up of sit-ups, stretches and pulling against towels (which is a waste of time, in case you've discovered these workouts on YouTube), then you won't be depleting your glucose or increasing your heartrate sufficiently to see results.

Instead, look for exercises that will provide a high enough intensity to get your heart rate to reach MHR. Remember: that is the whole *purpose* of a HIIT workout, so if it's not happening, you're not really doing HIIT.

Bodyweight lunges are not intensive unless you're in *particularly* bad shape, so instead try high knees, tuck jumps and kettlebell swings.

Remember that you can also increase your challenge by performing concurrent training. Kettlebell swings provide a great example of this but so too can various other challenges – like weighted pull-ups, or muscle-ups!

On the other end of the spectrum are those routines that are *too* challenging. While you might not like the idea of backing down from a workout, it's important to recognize that some routines are simply an invitation for injury. Chief among these are any routines that involve exhausting your cardiovascular system and then switching immediately to compound lifts with heavy weights. Do *not* exhaust yourself and then perform the muscle-up. The same goes for squats or deadlifts. These movements should go at the start of the circuit if you choose to include them and you should use a light(ish) weight to avoid injury. The more tired you get, the more your form will suffer. That doesn't matter for an incline press-up or a jumping jack, but it really *does* matter for a deadlift.

Another tip is to build the active recovery into your routine. If you can get your heartrate up to 95% MHR, then you can build in a small amount of active recovery at the next 30-second station. For example, you can perform tuck jumps followed by plank, or muscle-ups followed by light skipping. There will always be a station of *actual* recovery too though.

Finally, use other tricks to increase the calorie burn in a short space of time. If you switch from your legs to your upper body for example, then your heart will work harder in order to direct blood from top to bottom, as we discussed earlier.

Likewise, you can design your circuit with different lengths at each station in order to mimic something akin to cardio acceleration. Or why not use a long session of intense cardio right at the start of your circuit to increase the heart rate and reduce your glycogen stores? You can also add your own 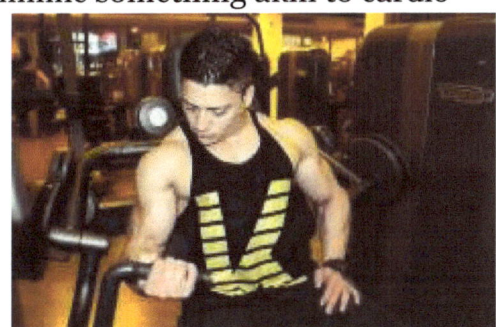 'finisher' at the end of your routines.

The best type of circuit routine if your aim is to burn fat and build muscle will be one that uses every muscle in the body. A whole body routine will not only provide the most 'even' improvements throughout your physique but will also help you to trigger the biggest release of growth hormone, testosterone and other anabolic hormones.

Building Muscle With Circuits

Want to build more size and less definition with your MetCon circuits? Then a good option is to use the same type of routine but to focus more on one muscle group.

For example, you might perform only bicep exercises as your main form of resistance training and schedule CV stations in between – essentially making a structured form of cardio acceleration.

This will then allow you to focus on one muscle group enough to cause *real* damage and metabolic stress. By continuously returning to the same muscle group, you'll be able to cause more microtears which will contribute to more repair and more growth/strength.

Likewise, you'll be able to flood that one muscle group with more blood and more hormones, which will make it more likely to grow in a very big way.

This now becomes something more akin to a bodybuilding workout but with the added cardio in order to provide the benefits of HIIT.

If you don't have time to focus each session on a different muscle group, then consider using a 'push pull' routine instead and switching between pushing movements and pulling movements to train the muscles.

Last Works: How to Add HIIT to a Healthy Lifestyle

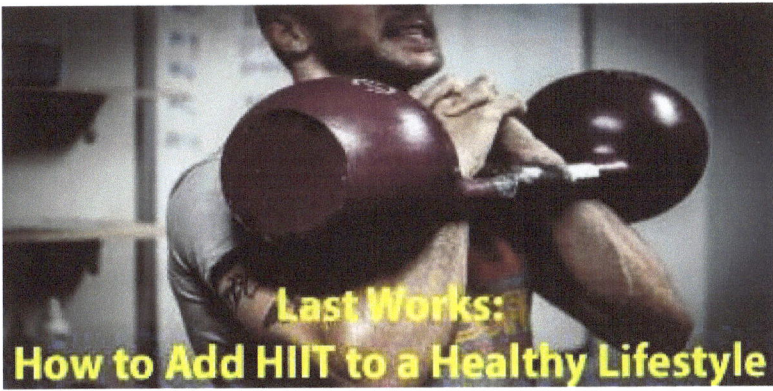

Hopefully this book has opened your eyes to the world of HIIT and just what a powerful training tool this really is. Moreover, I hope that you have discovered some new forms of HIIT and training that you might not have heard of before – and maybe you've learned that there's nothing wrong with creating your *own* protocols that are better suited to your goals. You know the science, so why not combine fartlek, cardio acceleration and MetCon into one brutal routine? Get inventive!

Before we go though, make sure you recognize the importance of combining your HIIT routines with the right lifestyle. If you want to maximize your fat loss and muscle building, then you should look at supplementing with extras like creatine and possibly a protein shake.

Losing weight also means eating a healthy diet that maintains a calorie deficit and if you want to avoid burning out, then you need to make sure you are getting plenty of rest and lots of sleep.

And don't throw the baby out with the bath water! HIIT is amazing, no doubt, but it's also only one piece of the puzzle.

Steady state cardio still has its advantages and is excellent for improving your resting heart rate for example. Likewise, you can use regular weight training in order to build muscle much quicker.

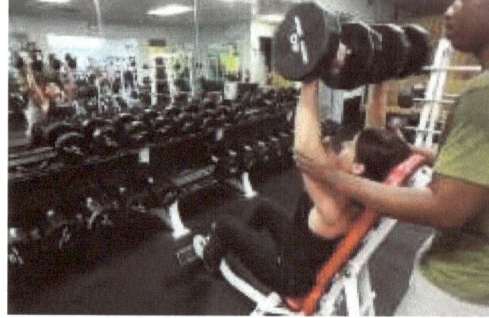

Instead of falling in love with each new training method and forgetting the old routines, instead look at how you can combine new information with what you already know to create something even more effective. How about using a Tabata routine at the end of your workouts as a finisher and throwing some steady state cardio into your routine as well?

Experiment and find what works for you. But the very last thing I want to leave you with is that you *must* make sure your routine is sustainable. Ask yourself honestly if the routine you've devised is something you can stick at indefinitely.

Remember: although HIIT is all about fits and starts, general health is a marathon, not a sprint.

Cheat Sheet

In this book, we looked at numerous different HIIT workouts and discussed a lot of the science and theory behind how they work. Hopefully, it has inspired you to start getting more creative with your workouts and to come up with some really challenging routines that will increase your strength, your fitness and your physique.

But it was a lot to take in all in one go. And with that in mind, this cheat sheet will provide you with a handy recap that you can dip into whenever you need a refresher, a little more inspiration or some new ideas!

The Three Energy Systems

The three energy systems are:

- The ATP-CP System: This stands for 'Adenosine Triphosphate Creatine Phosphate' system. This is the quickest energy system that the body has access to and it uses up energy stored inside the muscles in its most basic form. It can only last a few seconds, although creatine can enhance this slightly.

- The Glycogen Lactic Acid System: This is the second energy system. Once ATP-CP stores have been depleted in the muscle, the body will switch to the glycogen lactic acid system and this will use glycogen in the muscles. This can last for a couple of minutes but causes the build-up of metabolites in the muscle that cause the 'burn' sensation we associate with the gym. It also causes the build-up of lactic acid in the blood, which makes us feel nauseous and eventually forces us to reduce our activity.

- The Aerobic System: The last system that the body switches to is the aerobic system. Here, the heartrate works harder to pump oxygen to the fat stores. These get broken down and useable energy is then carried to the muscles to fuel movement. This can last indefinitely but puts the body in a highly catabolic state that breaks down muscle.

Types of HIIT

Regular HIIT: HIIT stands for 'High Intensity Interval Training' and the most basic form of this involves two intervals: a high intensity and low intensity interval. You then train at 90-100% of your maximum capacity for the fast interval and recover at around 70% for the slow interval. A starting ratio might be 30 seconds of high intensity and 2 minutes of low intensity. Eventually, you might end up doing 1 minute of high intensity and 1 minute of low!

Tabata: The tabata protocol is a highly popular HIIT workout that involves going all out for 20 seconds and then resting for 10 seconds. While 20 seconds might not seem like a long time, the short recovery periods mean that this can be absolutely brutal. The sequence is repeated 8 times, meaning that the entire thing lasts only 4 minutes – but is brilliant for burning a lot of fat.

Fartlek: Fartlek is a type of training that translates to 'time play'. The idea is that you're performing something akin to HIIT, except that you aren't switching between two different states but rather multiple states. What's more, is that you can choose how and when you make the change. You might then decide to walk for a period, jog for a while and then sprint. And you could mix those three states up in any way you choose – even in a non-linear or random fashion.

A great option is to sprint for 30 seconds and then go slower *until* your heartrate reaches a set point again to train your recovery.

MetCon: Speaking of training your recovery, MetCon is an abbreviation of 'Metabolic Conditioning' and is a type of training designed to improve your recovery and your energy efficiency. This often takes the form of circuits incorporating CV work and calisthenics. This can be used to tone and build muscle, while at the same time burning a lot of calories and improving fitness.

Advanced Concepts and Strategies

Cardio Acceleration: If you're feeling absolutely mad and you're willing to engage in a truly brutal workout, then consider 'cardio acceleration'. Here, you perform a regular weight lifting workout and use sets and repetitions of exercises. The difference is that you're not going to take the 1-minute rest in between as usual. Instead, you'll perform high intensity cardio in between each set. This will diminish your strength slightly but it also improves circulation and ensures that you're burning a huge number of calories for a resistance workout.

Concurrent Training: This simply means that you're combining both resistance work (such as weights) and cardio. An example is the kettlebell swing which can be performed for a long sequence but which requires you to move a heavy weight.

Concurrent training burns more calories than regular CV because it makes you use your fast twitch muscle fiber. At the same time, it also lets you increase the challenge for your muscles and stimulate growth.

This protects you against the muscle deterioration that can be caused by normal CV and it also makes your body more metabolically active subsequently.

Fasted Cardio: This is a type of cardio that you perform just before you have breakfast. This means that your body is in a fasted state as you won't have eaten during the night. By morning, you will have low blood sugar and low glycogen stores, meaning that your body has to work extra hard to get the energy it needs from fat. This has been shown to burn a lot more calories than regular exercise, though you should be cautious as it can also burn muscle.

Carb Backloading; Carb backloading is an eating strategy that involves eating right after you have engaged in high intensity exercise. This is a perfect match for your HIIT workouts, because it will allow you to direct the energy you consume to your muscles to restore glycogen stores *instead* of letting it be stored as fat. A lot of modern workout and diet regimes recommend that you only eat carbs after HIIT workouts and this is a very effective way to encourage weight loss. Definitely worth a try!

Mind Map

ATP-CP: Fast useable energy: stored as ATP in the muscles.
1-3 seconds
Glycogen Lactic Acid System: Fairly fast energy that causes a
build up of painful metabolites. Several minutes.
Aerobic Energy: Slowest system that burns fat using oxygen.
Indefinite

Kettlebells and battle ropes are ideal
for HIIT training thanks to their ability
to provide 'concurrent training' or
'resistance cardio'. You can train
your cardio fitness but while against
resistance.

The Energy Systems

Concurrent Training

Tabata

Tabata means:
20 seconds high intensity
10 seconds rest
8 rounds
Only for the experienced!

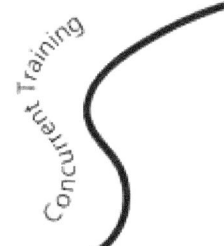

hiit workout

The Basics

Great HIIT Exercises

What is Metabolic Conditioning?

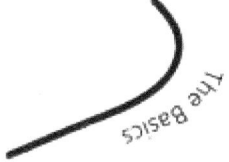

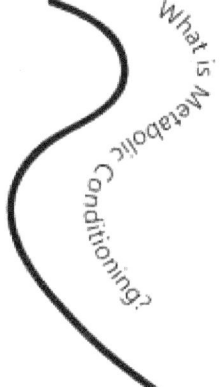

HIIT involves switching
from high intensity to low
intensity. This means you
are going from ATP-CP and
Glycogen LA to aerobic

You do this by training
at 90-100% MHR
(Max Heart Rate) for 30 seconds
to 2 minutes and switching
back to 70% for 1-3 minutes

This burns more calories in
less time and causes the
'afterburn effect'. It is great
for fitness and VO2 max.

* Kettlebell swing
* Running
* Cycling
* Swimming
* Punch bag
* Jump rope
* Rowing
* Battle ropes
* Calisthenics circuit
* Tuck jumps

Metabolic conditioning means
that you are using HIIT as part of
a resistance circuit. This is a great
way to build fitness while adding
muscle and losing fat.
Design your circuits smartly though
and think about sequencing!

Resources for Even Better Results

What's the secret to success with a good HIIT routine? The answer is that you design the routine sensibly and then give it 100% during your workouts.

But that's not to say that there aren't other factors that can also play a big role… and chief among these is the equipment you use. Read on and we'll look at some tools and supplements that can help you to get even more from your training.

Supplements

Nobody 'needs' supplements. However, they can certainly be beneficial and help you to see faster results and especially when choose the right supplements for your training.

There are a few that are ideally suited to HIIT…

Creatine: Creatine is the substance that the liver produces to recycle used ATP but you can also get it exogenously from your diet and from supplements. By being able to recycle ATP, creatine lets you use your ATP-CP system for a few seconds longer, thereby improving your ability to use high intensity training.

BCAAs: BCAAs are 'branch chained amino acids'. These are amino acids – the building blocks of proteins – that are in a more useable format. That is to say, that they are connected in a manner similar to the way they would need to be connected to become muscle. Studies show that when you consume BCAAs prior to a workout, they can help you to prevent muscle breakdown.

Preworkouts: Preworkouts are products designed to be

taken before a workout. They include BCAAs often but can also include other useful ingredients – such as stimulants like caffeine, bitter orange and l-carnitine to help increase your metabolism further!

Protein Shake: If you have any interest in building muscle as well as burning fat, you need extra protein. Protein shakes provide a great way to get this that is tasty and convenient. Just make sure you choose one that isn't packed with sugar and calories!

Tools

Running Trainers: If you're going to be running for your HIIT workouts, then running shoes are absolutely essential to allow you to avoid injury and to enjoy the ride.

Fitness Tracker: A fitness tracker has a ton of different advantages, from allowing you to monitor your calories burned throughout the day, to letting you check your heart rate in order to see how if your workouts are intense enough.

Heart Strap: Fitness trackers work best when paired with a heart rate monitor that is worn around the chest. Polar make some good models and these are more accurate than wrist-worn monitors.

Kettlebell: One of the most versatile pieces of training equipment in the world. The kettlebell is crucial for concurrent training and allows for extended periods of high effort work. The swing is an amazing movement that will melt calories and build your posterior chain.

Battle Ropes: Looking for another alternative form of cardio? Battle ropes are large heavy ropes that you hit against the ground quickly. This requires a lot of effort and once again is a generally excellent alternative to jogging or cycling.

Other Relevant Books by This Author

If you would like to read more relevant books about this topic, here is a list of the CreateSpace links, titles and descriptions from this author:

https://www.createspace.com/6516262

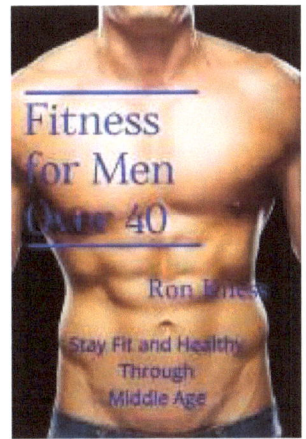

Fitness for Men Over 40: Stay Fit and Healthy Through Middle Age

A question I frequently hear asked is "Why do men over the age of 40 struggle to lose weight?" And it is a fair question.

That was about the time in my life when I had to start watching my weight. Now that I'm 65, it isn't getting any easier either as the years tick by. But with a lot of work, it is doable to keep your weight down and fitness level up. The chapters in this book show you how.

If you're a male in your forties or older, you definitely know the struggle is real. It doesn't matter if you were an athlete back in college or even a soldier back in the day as I was for 36 years … you will notice changes in your body.

You'll find it easier to gain weight and more difficult to lose it. If you do workout, you'll find it more difficult to do the same things you used to do with ease. The weights will seem heavier. Your stamina will have dropped.

You'll feel less energetic and driven.

The only consolation here is that whatever you may be feeling is very normal. It's part and parcel of aging. Let's look at why a man has a tougher time losing weight once he crosses forty.

In this book I'll show you what foods you should be eating and the exercise schedule you need to get and stay in shape as you continue through your middle age and into your senior years.

It is possible to get in shape or stay in shape as you continue to age.

https://www.createspace.com/6880021

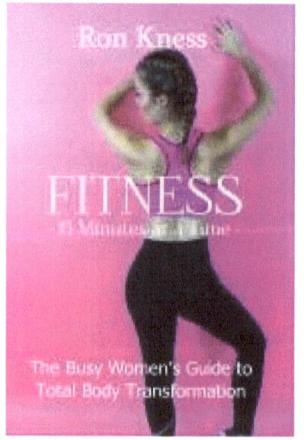

FITNESS - 15 Minutes at a TIme: The Busy Women's Guide to Total Body Transformation

We want to be healthier. We also want to be empowered with maintaining our weight and fitness level. And we want to keep the weight off and maintain our healthy lifestyle for the rest of our life!

We can achieve ALL of these goals with the newest release from Ron Kness called *Fitness 15 Minutes at a Time*. Based on these exciting teachings, you will learn about all the dramatic benefits of getting fit by eating healthy food resulting in weight loss, and doing high intensity exercising.

This book is built around a very clear, concept: improving your appearance and health.

It's not just about getting healthy. Having great fitness level is linked to reducing the risk of many diseases and even reversing the effects of some, such as being overweight and out of shape. These are just two of the many health benefits of being fit and at a normal weight.

In this book, we look at all the ways you can improve your own fitness level, starting with making the decision to get lose weight and healthy. That is the first step - you must want to do it!

This book also looks at the many other steps that can be taken to support this goal, from creating a calorie deficit - burning more calories than you eat - to exercising at a high intensity, to switching to a fitness and weight maintenance mode once at goal . The choices you make about the kind of food you eat and portion sizes has a big impact on your fitness level.

In *Fitness 15 Minutes at a Time*, we'll cover all the bases, giving you everything you need to know to eat healthy, lose weight and get fit.

https://www.createspace.com/6988627

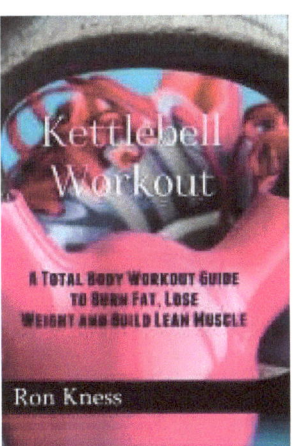

Kettlebell Workout: A Total Body Workout Guide to Burn Fat, Lose Weight and Build Lean Muscle

We want to be functionally stronger - that is building strength that we can use in our everyday lives. We also want to be in charge of our healthy lifestyle. And we want to use kettlebells safely as a workout program!

We can achieve ALL of these goals with the newest release from Ron Kness called *Kettlebell Workout - A Total Body Workout Guide To Burn Fat, Lose Weight And Build Lean Muscle.*

Based on these exciting teachings, you will learn about all the dramatic benefits of using kettlebells as exercise and proper nutrition as a way of getting healthy.

This book is built around a very clear, concept: burn fat, lose weight and build lean muscle.
It's not just about how to use kettlebells to burn fat, lose weight and build lean muscle. Having a great fitness level is linked to making smart exercise and nutrition decisions. This is because people living the healthy lifestyle have learned the value and benefits derived from being healthy.

In this book, we look at all of the ways you can improve your own fitness level, starting with strength training using kettlebells. This book will also look at the many other steps that can be taken to support this goal, from learning how to properly lift and swing kettlebells to torching calories from a kettlebell workout. The choices you make about healthy food and strength training has an impact on your fitness level.

In ***Kettlebell Workout - A Total Body Workout Guide To Burn Fat, Lose Weight And Build Lean Muscle***, we'll cover all the bases, giving you everything you need to know to properly use kettlebells as part of an overall fitness program.

About the Author

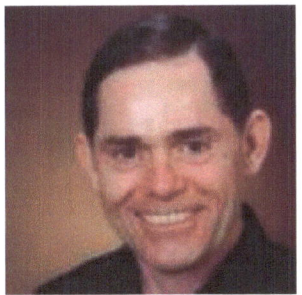

I have published over 125 books on Amazon for Kindle, CreateSpace and other publishing platforms.

While most of my books are on health and fitness in general, as I age (now 65) at the time of this writing) my topics of interest are geared toward aging baby boomers and older.

Besides my own writing, I also ghostwrite ebooks, books, reports, articles, blogs and do Kindle conversions for clients on a variety of topics.

Today my wife and I are retired from our careers and live in Gold Canyon, AZ. I now write as a retirement business where you'll find me happily sitting in my office typing away on my laptop as I work on my next book or ghostwriting project . . . that is if we are not traveling on a cruise ship - our new-found mode of travel.

www.ingramcontent.com/pod-product-compliance
Lightning Source LLC
Chambersburg PA
CBHW050816290526
45792CB00001B/140